Pharmacy Law Quizzes: 2nd Edition

By Babir Malik

Text copyright © 2022 Babir Malik
All Rights Reserved

About the author

Babir studied pharmacy at the University of Bradford and graduated in 2007 (after previously studying Biomedical Sciences at the same university). He joined Weldricks Pharmacy as a summer student in 2005, undertook his pre-reg with them and has stayed with them ever since.

Babir is now the Weldricks Foundation and Pharmacy Student Lead and also an Assistant Professor in Pharmacy Practice at the University of Bradford. He is also the Green Light Campus Foundation Quality Assurance Lead, Charity Ambassador for Pharmacist Support, and Associate Fellow at HEA.

Babir currently practices as a relief pharmacist for Weldricks on Saturday mornings. In June 2016, the pharmacy that he co-managed at the time was awarded the Chemist and Druggist Medicines Optimisation Award for their innovative Local Pharmaceutical Service Intervention Service. He is a Chemist and Druggist Clinical Advisory Board Member.

He is also the MPharm Calculations Lead at the University of Bradford. Furthermore, Babir undertook a 10-week secondment as a Clinical Commissioning Group Pharmacist in North Lincolnshire early in 2016. He is also on the Medicines, Ethics and Practice Advisory Group. He completed his Clinical Diploma in Community Pharmacy at the University of Keel and is an RPS Fellow.

He can be found quite often on Twitter @Babir1981

Preface

I am delighted to share with you the second edition of Pharmacy Law Quizzes. The first edition was warmly received in 2020. This edition is in the style of flashcards with each question on one page and the answer on the next page.

While Pharmacy Law is not always the most exciting of topics it is a vital part of pharmacy, especially community pharmacy.

This book should be used after you have read the MEP or your lecture notes and before attempting law multiple choice questions. It is also a fun way of refreshing your knowledge as pharmacist or pharmacy technician and could be used as tool to aid revision for the registration assessment.

This book is not endorsed by the Royal Pharmaceutical Society or General Pharmaceutical Council or any organisation that I work for.

This book was written using MEP 45 and was correct at the time of publication. There are no worked answers and if you are unsure after seeing the correct answer then please refer to the latest MEP.

If you have any comments, questions, or suggestions for topics then I can be contacted on
pharmacylawquizzes@gmail.com

Babir

Foreword

I first bumped into Babir almost 7 years ago at a pre-registration (now foundation) careers fair. He was there to showcase what his organisation had to offer as part of their training programme. Over the years I have not seen any individual dedicate so much of their own time to support trainees and students who are not his responsibility. Weekends, evenings, online groups, Zoom calls, workshops - the list goes on.

In addition to how generous Babir is with his time, the one thing that has really struck me is his attention to detail when it comes to all matters relating to pharmacy practice. There are many people out there attempting to support trainees, but very few have the eye for detail and keep abreast of developments as sharply as Babir does.

This latest edition of Pharmacy Law Quizzes is a great tool to reinforce your knowledge of pharmacy law. Obviously, this is important for anyone preparing for an assessment, but more importantly it's vital to understand the law to keep you on the register. I spent 4 years on the GPhC Fitness to Practice Committee observing some of the weird and wonderful things our colleagues get up to - this book should help prevent you becoming an anecdote in a school of pharmacy lecture theatre!

Khalid Khan

Head of Training & Professional Standards
Imaan Healthcare

Acknowledgements

I would like to thank Joanna Jamroz, Klaudia Zelanzy and Raffaella Woolmer for their kind assistance.

Glossary

CD: Controlled drugs
EEA: European Economic Area
EHC: Emergency Hormonal Contraception
GMC: General Medical Council
GSL: General Sales List
HMR 2012: Human Medicines Regulation 2012
MEP: Medicines, Ethics and Practice
MHRA: Medicines and Healthcare products Regulatory Agency
NFA-VPS: Non-Food Animal – Veterinarian, Pharmacist, Suitably Qualified Person
OTC: Over the Counter
P: Pharmacy medicine
PGD: Patient Group Direction.
POM: Prescription-only Medicine
POM-V: Prescription-only Medicine – Veterinarian
POM-VPS: Prescription-only Medicine – Veterinarian, Pharmacist, Suitably Qualified Person
PPP: Pregnancy Prevention Programme
PSD: Patient Specific Direction
RP: Responsible Pharmacist
RPS: Royal Pharmaceutical Society

1. A no-blame culture is better than a punitive or just culture: **True or False?**

A no-blame culture is better than a punitive or just culture: **False**

?

2. Poor growth and weight of a child can be a sign of neglect: **True or False?**

Poor growth and weight of a child can be a sign of neglect:
True

?

3. Getting into debt could be a sign of financial abuse in a vulnerable adult: **True or False?**

Getting into debt could be a sign of financial abuse in a vulnerable adult: **True**

4. There are five principles of medicines optimisation: **True or False?**

There are five principles of medicines optimisation: **False**

?

5. Medicines account for about 25% of carbon emissions within the NHS: **True or False?**

Medicines account for about 25% of carbon emissions within the NHS: True

?

6. There are two classes of medicinal products for humans under the Human Medicines Regulations 2012: **True or False?**

There are two classes of medicinal products for humans under the Human Medicines Regulations 2012:
False

7. GSL medicines can only be sold from a pharmacy: **True or False?**

GSL medicines can only be sold from a pharmacy: **False**

?

8. P medicines can be available for self-selection: **True or False?**

P medicines can be available for self-selection: **False**

9. A physiotherapist independent prescriber can prescribe schedule 2 CDs: **True or False?**

A physiotherapist independent prescriber can prescribe schedule 2 CDs: **True**

10. It is unlawful to sell a product that contains more than 600mg of pseudoephedrine: **True or False?**

It is unlawful to sell a product that contains more than 600mg of pseudoephedrine: **False**

11. It is unlawful to sell a product that contains more than 180mg of ephedrine: **True or False?**

It is unlawful to sell a product that contains more than 180mg of ephedrine: True

12. It is unlawful to sell a pseudoephedrine product at the same time as an ephedrine product: **True or False?**

It is unlawful to sell a pseudoephedrine product at the same time as an ephedrine product: **True**

13. There are two methods of emergency contraception: **True or False?**

There are two methods of emergency contraception: **False**

14. Advanced supply of EHC is allowed:
True or False?

Advanced supply of EHC is allowed: **True**

15. Ulipristal acetate is only licensed for emergency contraception within 72 hours of unprotected sexual intercourse: **True or False?**

Ulipristal acetate is only licensed for emergency contraception within 72 hours of unprotected sexual intercourse: **False**

16. Ulipristal acetate is licensed from 14 years of age: **True or False?**

Ulipristal acetate is licensed from 14 years of age: **False**

17. Levonorgestrel is only licensed for emergency contraception within 120 hours of unprotected sexual intercourse: **True or False?**

Levonorgestrel is only licensed for emergency contraception within 120 hours of unprotected sexual intercourse: **False**

18. The legal limit of paracetamol effervescent tablets that can be sold is 100: **True or False?**

The legal limit of paracetamol effervescent tablets that can be sold is 100: **False**

19. The maximum pack size for OTC dihydrocodeine is 16: **True or False?**

The maximum pack size for OTC dihydrocodeine is 16: **False**

20. OTC co-codamol cannot be sold for a sore throat: **True or False?**

OTC co-codamol cannot be sold for a sore throat:
True

21. NHS and private prescriptions have different legal requirements: **True or False?**

NHS and private prescriptions have different legal requirements: **False**

22. The date of birth is a legal requirement on a prescription for a POM: **True or False?**

The date of birth is a legal requirement on a prescription for a POM:
False

23. The name of the prescriber is a legal requirement on a prescription: **True or False?**

The name of the prescriber is a legal requirement on a prescription: **False**

24. If a patient is under 12, then there is a legal requirement for their age to be stated on the prescription: **True or False?**

If a patient is under 12, then there is a legal requirement for their age to be stated on the prescription: **True**

?

25. All prescriptions are valid for up to 6 months from the appropriate date: **True or False?**

All prescriptions are valid for up to 6 months from the appropriate date:
False

?

26. It is not a legal requirement for all prescriptions to be written in English: **True or False?**

It is not a legal requirement for all prescriptions to be written in English: **True**

27. Private prescriptions for Schedule 4 and 5 CDs cannot be repeated: **True or False?**

Private prescriptions for Schedule 4 and 5 CDs cannot be repeated:
False

?

28. The first dispensing of a private prescription must be made within 6 months of the appropriate date, following which there is no legal time limit for the remaining repeats: **True or False?**

The first dispensing of a private prescription must be made within 6 months of the appropriate date, following which there is no legal time limit for the remaining repeats: **True**

29. NHS prescriptions can be repeated: **True or False?**

NHS prescriptions can be repeated: **False**

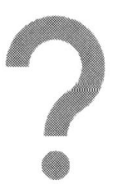

30. Owings for co-codamol 30/500 tablets are valid for 28 days from the appropriate date: **True or False?**

Owings for co-codamol 30/500 tablets are valid for 28 days from the appropriate date: **False**

?

31. The name of the drug is a legal requirement for a POM: **True or False?**

The name of the drug is a legal requirement for a POM: **False**

?

32. The quantity of the drug is a legal requirement for a POM: **True or False?**

The quantity of the drug is a legal requirement for a POM: **False**

33. Private prescriptions for a POM must be retained for 2 years after dispensing: **True or False?**

Private prescriptions for a POM must be retained for 2 years after dispensing:
True

34. Repeat slips are not prescriptions: **True or False?**

Repeat slips are not prescriptions: **True**

?

35. If the number of repeats is not stated on a private prescription, it can only be dispensed twice: **True or False?**

If the number of repeats is not stated on a private prescription, it can only be dispensed twice: **True**

36. Private prescriptions for oral contraceptives are exempt from record keeping: **True or False?**

Private prescriptions for oral contraceptives are exempt from record keeping: **True**

?

37. The dose is a legal requirement when making a private prescription record in the POM register: **True or False?**

The dose is a legal requirement when making a private prescription record in the POM register: **False**

38. Schedule 2, 3, 4 and 5 CD Owings are valid for 28 days after the appropriate date: **True or False?**

Schedule 2, 3, 4 and 5 CD Owings are valid for 28 days after the appropriate date: **False**

39. Electronic prescriptions must still meet the general prescription requirements: **True or False?**

Electronic prescriptions must still meet the general prescription requirements: **True**

40. Faxed prescriptions are legal: **True or False?**

Faxed prescriptions are legal: **False**

?

41. Dentists are only legally allowed to prescribe medicines on the Dental Practitioners Formulary: **True or False?**

Dentists are only legally allowed to prescribe medicines on the Dental Practitioners Formulary:
False

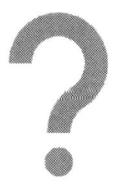

42. If "Dr" appears before the prescriber signature, then it could be a forged prescription: **True or False?**

If "Dr" appears before the prescriber signature, then it could be a forged prescription: **True**

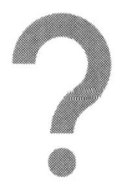

43. A patient's date of birth is a legal requirement on an EEA prescription: **True or False?**

A patient's date of birth is a legal requirement on an EEA prescription: **True**

44. The name of the prescriber is a legal requirement on an EEA prescription: **True or False?**

The name of the prescriber is a legal requirement on an EEA prescription: **True**

?

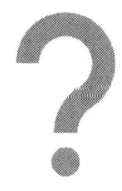

45. EEA Prescriptions must be written in English: **True or False?**

EEA Prescriptions must be written in English:
False

46. The prescriber's email address is a legal requirement on an EEA prescription: **True or False?**

The prescriber's email address is a legal requirement on an EEA prescription: True

?

47. The name of the drug is a legal requirement on an EEA prescription: **True or False?**

The prescriber's email address is a legal requirement on an EEA prescription: **True**

48. EEA prescriptions are subject to prescription charges: **True or False?**

EEA prescriptions are subject to prescription charges: **False**

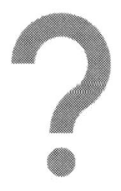

49. Schedule 1, 2 and 3 CDs are not allowed on an EEA prescription: **True or False?**

Schedule 1, 2 and 3 CDs are not allowed on an EEA prescription: **True**

50. Medicinal products without a marketing authorisation valid in the UK are not allowed on an EEA prescription: **True or False?**

Medicinal products without a marketing authorisation valid in the UK are not allowed on an EEA prescription: **True**

51. Emergency supply at the request of an EEA prescriber is allowed: **True or False?**

Emergency supply at the request of an EEA prescriber is allowed:

True

☐

52. Emergency supply at the request of an EEA patient for phenobarbital for epilepsy is allowed: **True or False?**

Emergency supply at the request of an EEA patient for phenobarbital for epilepsy is allowed: **False**

53. It is a legal requirement for the name of the doctor to appear on a dispensing label: **True or False?**

It is a legal requirement for the name of the doctor to appear on a dispensing label: **False**

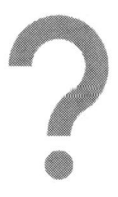

54. It is a legal requirement for the date of dispensing to appear on a dispensing label: **True or False?**

It is a legal requirement for the date of dispensing to appear on a dispensing label: **True**
☐

55. Additional information can be added to the dispensing label if the pharmacist considers it to be necessary: **True or False?**

Additional information can be added to the dispensing label if the pharmacist considers it to be necessary: **True**

56. A patient specific direction is a written direction that allows the supply and/or administration of a specified medicine or medicines, by named authorised health professionals, to a well-defined group of patients requiring treatment for a specific condition: **True or False?**

A patient specific direction is a written direction that allows the supply and/or administration of a specified medicine or medicines, by named authorised health professionals, to a well-defined group of patients requiring treatment for a specific condition: **False**

?

57. Regulation 238 of HMR 2012 allows insulin to be administered by anyone for the purpose of saving life in an emergency: **True or False?**

Regulation 238 of HMR 2012 allows insulin to be administered by anyone for the purpose of saving life in an emergency:
False

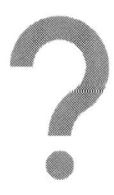

58. In an emergency, a pharmacist working in a registered pharmacy can supply POMs to an animal without a prescription: **True or False?**

In an emergency, a pharmacist working in a registered pharmacy can supply POMs to an animal without a prescription: **False**

?

59. A podiatrist independent prescriber can request an emergency supply: **True or False?**

A podiatrist independent prescriber can request an emergency supply: **True**

?

60. A paramedic independent prescriber can request an emergency supply: **True or False?**

A paramedic independent prescriber can request an emergency supply: **True**

?

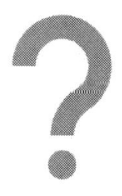

61. In an emergency supply at the request of a prescriber, the prescriber must furnish a prescription within 48 hours: **True or False?**

In an emergency supply at the request of a prescriber, the prescriber must furnish a prescription within 48 hours: **False**

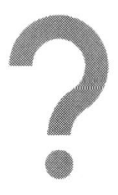

62. In an emergency supply at the request of a prescriber, the prescriber can only authorise a maximum of 30 days' supply for POMs: **True or False?**

In an emergency supply at the request of a prescriber, the prescriber can only authorise a maximum of 30 days' supply for POMs: **False**

63. When making a POM register entry for an emergency supply at a request of a prescriber, two dates should be entered: **True or False?**

When making a POM register entry for an emergency supply at a request of a prescriber, two dates should be entered: **False**

?

64. Legislation prevents a pharmacist from making an emergency supply when the doctor's surgery is open: **True or False?**

Legislation prevents a pharmacist from making an emergency supply when the doctor's surgery is open: **False**

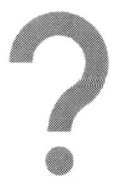

65. An emergency supply of phenobarbital in the UK can only be supplied for a maximum of 5 days: **True or False?**

An emergency supply of phenobarbital in the UK can only be supplied for a maximum of 5 days: **True**

?

66. When making a POM register entry for emergency supply at the request of a prescriber, the dose is a legal requirement: **True or False?**

When making a POM register entry for emergency supply at the request of a prescriber, the dose is a legal requirement: **False**

67. All optometrists and podiatrists can authorise supplies of POMs by writing prescriptions: **True or False?**

All optometrists and podiatrists can authorise supplies of POMs by writing prescriptions:
False

?

68. Schools can obtain beclometasone and salbutamol inhalers via a signed order: **True or False?**

Schools can obtain beclometasone and salbutamol inhalers via a signed order: **False**

?

69. Any schoolteacher can sign a signed order to obtain salbutamol inhalers: **True or False?**

Any schoolteacher can sign a signed order to obtain salbutamol inhalers: **False**

70. The names of the students needing the salbutamol inhalers should be on the signed order: **True or False?**

The names of the students needing the salbutamol inhalers should be on the signed order: **False**

?

71. A maximum of five salbutamol inhalers can be supplied to a school on a signed order: **True or False?**

A maximum of five salbutamol inhalers can be supplied to a school on a signed order: **False**

72. Appropriately headed paper must be used on a signed order for adrenaline auto-injectors for a school: **True or False?**

Appropriately headed paper must be used on a signed order for adrenaline auto-injectors for a school: **False**

73. Any pharmacist can supply nasal naloxone to a substance misuser without a prescription, PSD or PGD: **True or False?**

Any pharmacist can supply nasal naloxone to a substance misuser without a prescription, PSD or PGD: **False**

?

74. All women wanting isotretinoin prescriptions must comply with PPP: **True or False?**

All women wanting isotretinoin prescriptions must comply with the PPP: **False**

?

75. Under the PPP, prescriptions for acitretin are valid for 7 days: **True or False?**

Under the PPP, prescriptions for acitretin are valid for 7 days: **True**

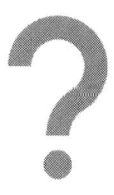

76. All prescriptions for isotretinoin should only be prescribed for 30 days: **True or False?**

All prescriptions for isotretinoin should only be prescribed for 30 days: **False**

77. Pharmacists should not accept repeat prescriptions for oral retinoids: **True or False?**

Pharmacists should not accept repeat prescriptions for oral retinoids: **True**

78. Under the PPP, prescriptions for valproate are valid for 7 days: **True or False?**

Under the PPP, prescriptions for valproate are valid for 7 days: **False**

79. Those planning pregnancies and taking valproate must schedule an appointment with their prescriber and stop taking valproate immediately: **True or False?**

Those planning pregnancies and taking valproate must schedule an appointment with their prescriber and stop taking valproate immediately: **False**

80. When dispensing valproate, pharmacists should ensure that a patient card is provided every time: **True or False?**

When dispensing valproate, pharmacists should ensure that a patient card is provided every time: **True**

81. All biologics should be prescribed by brand: **True or False?**

All biologics should be prescribed by brand:
True

☐

82. Lantus is an example of an original biologic medicine: **True or False?**

Lantus is an example of an original biologic medicine: **True**

83. A Pharmacist Independent Prescriber can prescribe unlicensed medicines subject to accepted good clinical practice: **True or False?**

A Pharmacist Independent Prescriber can prescribe unlicensed medicines subject to accepted good clinical practice: **True**

?

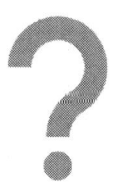

84. An optometrist independent prescriber can authorise an emergency supply for items that they can prescribe: **True or False?**

An optometrist independent prescriber can authorise an emergency supply for items that they can prescribe: **True**

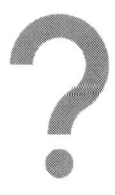

85. A Vet can authorise an emergency supply for items that they can prescribe: **True or False?**

A Vet can authorise an emergency supply for items that they can prescribe: **False**

?

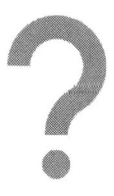

86. Pharmacies can supply appropriate health professionals with a small number of POMs via wholesale dealing if only a small profit is made: **True or False?**

Pharmacies can supply appropriate health professionals with a small number of POMs via wholesale dealing if only a small profit is made:
False

87. An independent nurse prescriber can be supplied with a small number of medicines via wholesale dealing: **True or False?**

An independent nurse prescriber can be supplied with a small number of medicines via wholesale dealing: **False**

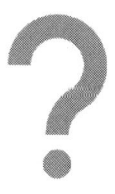

88. POM-VPS are prescription-only medicines that can only be prescribed by a Vet and supplied by a Vet or pharmacist with a written prescription: **True or False?**

POM-VPS are prescription-only medicines that can only be prescribed by a Vet and supplied by a Vet or pharmacist with a written prescription: **False**

89. A written prescription is needed to supply an NFA-VPS medicine: **True or False?**

A written prescription is needed to supply an NFA-VPS medicine:
False

90. Vet prescriptions for Schedule 2, 3 and 4 drugs are valid for 28 days: **True or False?**

Vet prescriptions for Schedule 2, 3 and 4 drugs are valid for 28 days: **True**

91. The Veterinary Medicines Directorate advise that "as directed" is a legally acceptable dosage instruction on a vet prescription: **True or False?**

The Veterinary Medicines Directorate advise that "as directed" is a legally acceptable dosage instruction on a vet prescription: **False**

92. Standardised forms are required for Vet schedule 2 and 3 CD prescriptions:
True or False?

Standardised forms are required for Vet schedule 2 and 3 CD prescriptions:
False

93. Vet CD prescriptions should be sent to the relevant NHS agency: **True or False?**

Vet CD prescriptions should be sent to the relevant NHS agency:
False

94. For all CDs, it is considered good practice for only 28 days' worth of treatment to be prescribed on a vet prescription: **True or False?**

For all CDs, it is considered good practice for only 28 days' worth of treatment to be prescribed on a vet prescription: **True**

?

95. All vet prescriptions must include the Royal College of Veterinary Surgeons Registration number of the Vet: **True or False?**

All vet prescriptions must include the Royal College of Veterinary Surgeons Registration number of the Vet: **False**

?

96. The cascade exemption within the Veterinary Medicines Regulations allows the supply of medicines that are not licensed for animals: **True or False?**

The cascade exemption within the Veterinary Medicines Regulations allows the supply of medicines that are not licensed for animals:
True

?

97. It is lawful to sell human medicines for use in animals: **True or False?**

It is lawful to sell human medicines for use in animals: **False**

?

98. The expiry date of a medicine supplied under the cascade must always be on the dispensing label: **True or False?**

The expiry date of a medicine supplied under the cascade must always be on the dispensing label: **False**

?

99. An entry must be made in the POM register for all POM-V and POM-VPS: **True or False?**

An entry must be made in the POM register for all POM-V and POM-VPS: **False**

100. Register entries for POM-V and POM-VPS can be kept electronically: **True or False?**

Register entries for POM-V and POM-VPS can be kept electronically: **True**

?

101. Records and documents for POM-V and POM-VPS must be kept for two years: **True or False?**

Records and documents for POM-V and POM-VPS must be kept for two years: **False**

102. Animal adverse reactions and human adverse reactions to vet medicines should be reported to the MHRA: **True or False?**

Animal adverse reactions and human adverse reactions to vet medicines should be reported to the MHRA:
False

103. NFA-VPS medicines should not be accessible by the public in a pharmacy: **True or False?**

NFA-VPS medicines should not be accessible by the public in a pharmacy: True

104. The Health Act 2006 introduced the concept of an accountable officer:
True or False?

The Health Act 2006 introduced the concept of an accountable officer:
True

?

105. There are two classes of Schedule 5 drugs: **True or False?**

There are two classes of Schedule 5 drugs: **True**

?

106. Dexamfetamine is a Schedule 2 drug:
True or False?

Dexamfetamine is a Schedule 2 drug: **True**

?

107. Temazepam has safe custody requirements: **True or False?**

Temazepam has safe custody requirements:
True

?

108. Morphine is only a Schedule 2 drug:
True or False?

Morphine is only a Schedule 2 drug: **False**

?

109. Entries should be made in the CD register for buprenorphine: **True or False?**

Entries should be made in the CD register for buprenorphine: **False**

?

110. Entries should be made in the CD register for pethidine: **True or False?**

Entries should be made in the CD register for pethidine: **True**

111. Sativex is a Schedule 4 Part II CD: **True or False?**

Sativex is a Schedule 4 Part II CD: **False**

112. Nabilone is a Schedule 2 CD: **True or False?**

Nabilone is a Schedule 2 CD: **False**

113. Epidyolex is a Schedule 5 CD: **True or False?**

Epidyolex is a Schedule 5 CD: True

☐

114. Dronabinol is a Schedule 2 CD: **True or False?**

Dronabinol is a Schedule 2 CD: **True**

?

115. Prescriptions for zopiclone are only valid for 28 days after the appropriate date: **True or False?**

Prescriptions for zopiclone are only valid for 28 days after the appropriate date: True

116. The address of prescriber for a schedule 4 CD must be in the UK: **True or False?**

The address of prescriber for a schedule 4 CD must be in the UK: **False**

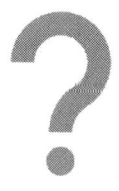

117. NICE advise that organisations should consider retaining all CD invoices for six years for the purposes of HM Revenue and Customs: **True or False?**

NICE advise that organisations should consider retaining all CD invoices for six years for the purposes of HM Revenue and Customs:
True

?

118. Pharmacists can, under one specific exemption, take possession of a schedule 1 CD: **True or False?**

Pharmacists can, under one specific exemption, take possession of a schedule 1 CD: **False**

119. The name of supplier is a legal requirement for a CD requisition: **True or False?**

The name of supplier is a legal requirement for a CD requisition: **False**

120. The total quantity of a drug in words and figures is a legal requirement for a CD requisition: **True or False?**

The total quantity of a drug in words and figures is a legal requirement for a CD requisition: **False**

121. There are six legal requirements for a CD requisition: **True or False?**

There are six legal requirements for a CD requisition: **True**

122. In an emergency, a doctor or dentist can be supplied with a Schedule 2 or 3 CD on the undertaking that a requisition will be supplied within the next 24 hours: **True or False?**

In an emergency, a doctor or dentist can be supplied with a Schedule 2 or 3 CD on the undertaking that a requisition will be supplied within the next 24 hours: **True**

123. When a requisition for a schedule 1, 2 or 3 CD is received, it is a legal requirement to mark the requisition indelibly with the supplier's name and address: **True or False?**

When a requisition for a schedule 1, 2 or 3 CD is received, it is a legal requirement to mark the requisition indelibly with the supplier's name and address: **True**

?

124. The person requesting the CD must send the original requisition to the relevant NHS agency: **True or False?**

The person requesting the CD must send the original requisition to the relevant NHS agency:
False

125. A registered midwife may use a midwife supply order to obtain diamorphine, morphine, and oxycodone: **True or False?**

A registered midwife may use a midwife supply order to obtain diamorphine, morphine, and oxycodone: **False**

?

126. The name of prescriber is a legal requirement on a prescription for a schedule 2 or 3 CD: **True or False?**

The name of prescriber is a legal requirement on a prescription for a schedule 2 or 3 CD:
False

127. The dose on a schedule 2 or 3 CD prescription does not need to be in words and figures: **True or False?**

The dose on a schedule 2 or 3 CD prescription does not need to be in words and figures: **True**

?

128. The name of drug is not a legal requirement on a schedule 2 or 3 CD prescription: **True or False?**

The name of drug is not a legal requirement on a schedule 2 or 3 CD prescription: True

129. "No fixed Abode" is acceptable as the address on a CD prescription: **True or False?**

"No fixed Abode" is acceptable as the address on a CD prescription: **True**

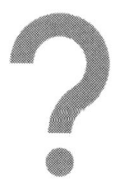

130. It is a legal requirement for schedule 2, 3 or 4 CD prescriptions to not exceed a 30-day supply: **True or False?**

It is a legal requirement for schedule 2, 3 or 4 CD prescriptions to not exceed a 30-day supply:
False

?

131. An independent nurse prescriber can prescribe methadone for addiction: **True or False?**

An independent nurse prescriber can prescribe methadone for addiction:
True

?

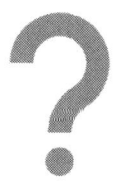

132. When a schedule 2 or 3 CD is supplied, it is a requirement to mark the prescription with the date of supply at the time the supply is made: **True or False?**

When a schedule 2 or 3 CD is supplied, it is a requirement to mark the prescription with the date of supply at the time the supply is made: **True**

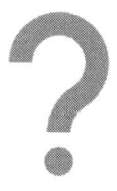

133. The GMC number of a prescriber must be included on a private CD prescription: **True or False?**

The GMC number of a prescriber must be included on a private CD prescription: **False**

134. Day 1 of 28 days validity for a Schedule 2 prescription starts the day after the prescription is signed: **True or False?**

Day 1 of 28 days validity for a Schedule 2 prescription starts the day after the prescription is signed: **True**

135. Supervision on an instalment prescription is a legal requirement: **True or False?**

Supervision on an instalment prescription is a legal requirement:
False

136. A pharmacist may request evidence of that person's identity if not already known to them when dispensing a schedule 2 or 3 CD prescription: **True or False?**

A pharmacist may request evidence of that person's identity if not already known to them when dispensing a schedule 2 or 3 CD prescription: **False**

137. Midazolam and phenobarbital are not subject to safe custody: **True or False?**

Midazolam and phenobarbital are not subject to safe custody:
True

?

138. For patient returned CDs an entry must be made in the CD register: **True or False?**

For patient returned CDs an entry must be made in the CD register: **False**

?

139. For CDs supplied, the name of the pharmacist supplying must be recorded in the CD register: **True or False?**

For CDs supplied, the name of the pharmacist supplying must be recorded in the CD register: **False**

?

140. CD register entries must be made on the day of supply: **True or False?**

CD register entries must be made on the day of supply: **False**

?

141. A CD running balance is not a legal requirement: **True or False?**

A CD running balance is not a legal requirement:
True

142. A statutory medical defence can be raised if driving is impaired and a specific drug is detected at higher levels than those permitted in the regulations, if there is evidence that the drug has been prescribed or bought and taken in accordance with the patient information leaflet: **True or False?**

A statutory medical defence can be raised if driving is impaired and a specific drug is detected at higher levels than those permitted in the regulations, if there is evidence that the drug has been prescribed or bought and taken in accordance with the patient information leaflet: **False**

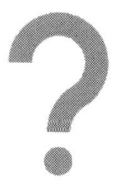

143. The pharmacist's RPS number must be displayed on the RP notice: **True or False?**

The pharmacist's RPS number must be displayed on the RP notice: **False**

?

144. The pharmacy record can be in writing, electronic or both: **True or False?**

The pharmacy record can be in writing, electronic or both: **True**

?

145. The reason for any absence by the RP must be stated in the RP record: **True or False?**

The reason for any absence by the RP must be stated in the RP record: **False**

?

146. The RP must personally make entries in the RP record: **True or False?**

The RP must personally make entries in the RP record: **True**

?

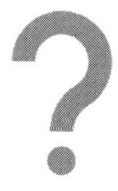

147. If two pharmacists are working together, both can be RP at the same time: **True or False?**

If two pharmacists are working together, both can be RP at the same time: **False**

148. GSL medicines can be sold in the absence of an RP but only if the RP is signed in: **True or False?**

GSL medicines can be sold in the absence of an RP but only if the RP is signed in: **True**

?

149. Explicit and implied consent are the two types of consent: **True or False?**

Explicit and implied consent are the two types of consent: **True**

150. Ordering stock from wholesalers can take place without an RP in charge of the pharmacy: **True or False?**

Ordering stock from wholesalers can take place without an RP in charge of the pharmacy: True

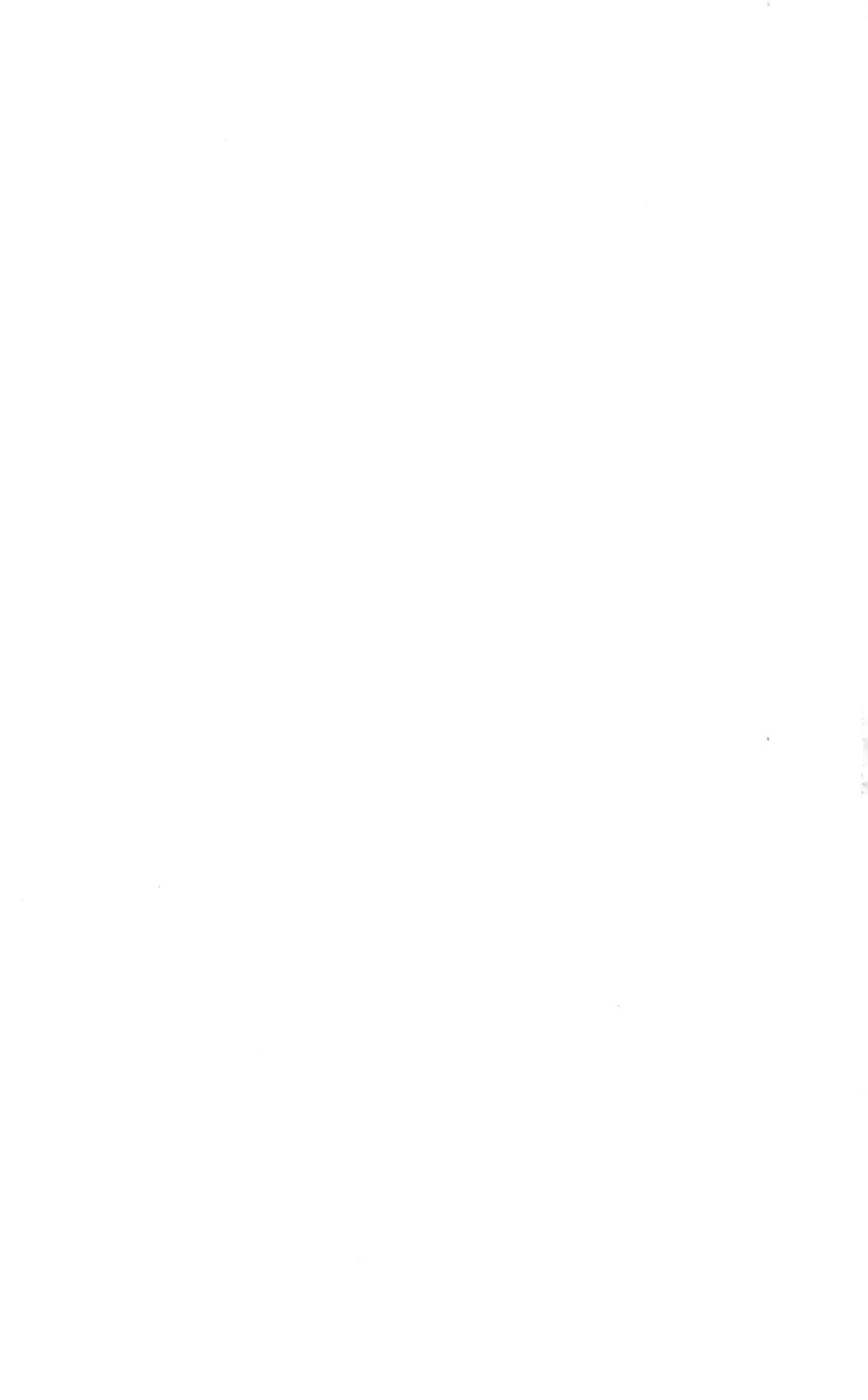

Printed in Great Britain
by Amazon